The Esser
Mediterranean
Diet Cookbook

Simple and Affordable Recipes from the World Healthiest Cuisine

Debbie Gillian

TABLE OF CONTANTS

INTRODUCTION

The Mediterranean diet is an eating way that is naturally low in processed foods and added sugar. Mediterranean Diet is based on fresh fruits and vegetables, whole grains, unsaturated fats, and fish instead of meat. It's about keeping things simple and healthy and that's why it's been around for so long. A study conducted at the University of Crete Medical School in Greece found that the Mediterranean diet can reduce the risk of premature death by 40 percent. The study followed the health outcomes of 20,000 participants, aged 55 and older, over a six-year period.

In fact, the Italian Mediterranean diet is one of the very first and most popular diets in the world today, as it has been proven to be a great, healthy diet. Indeed, the Italian Mediterranean diet changes the way people view dieting and adhering to a strict diet plan. Be as it may, there is a lot more to the diet plan than merely following a strict diet plan, and sticking to it will undoubtedly be enough to keep one fit and healthy.

The dietary pattern is connected through reductions of all-cause mortality in observational studies. There is also some indication that the Mediterranean diet decreases the risk of heart failure and early death; that is why the American Medical Association and the (AHA) American Heart Association suggest this diet.

Though there are many opposing views on the Mediterranean diet, some controversy over some sources says that the Italian Mediterranean diet is actually not that great because there are numerous other diets similar in style to that.

It has been proven to be an excellent way of maintaining health and living a long, healthy life. Still, the Italian Mediterranean diet is an excellent way of living and has been proven to produce great results. It is undoubtedly a great diet plan to follow. The Italian Mediterranean diet can also create long-term effects in keeping one's heart-healthy and body functioning at optimum levels.

BREAKFAST RECIPES

1. Ham Muffins

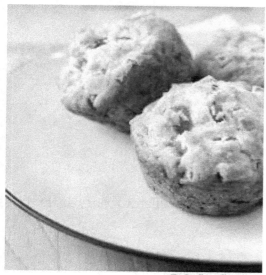

HankysHappyHome.com

Preparation Time: 10 Minutes

Cooking Time: 15 minutes

Servings: 4

Ingredients

- 3 oz ham, chopped

- 4 eggs, beaten

- 2 tablespoons coconut flour

- ½ teaspoon dried oregano

- ¼ teaspoon dried cilantro

Directions

1.   Spray the muffin's molds with cooking spray from inside.

2.   In the bowl mix up together beaten eggs, coconut flour, dried oregano, cilantro, and ham.

3.   When the liquid is homogenous, pour it in the prepared muffin molds.

4.   Bake the muffins for 15 minutes at 360F.

5.   Chill the cooked meal well and only after this remove from the molds.

Nutrition: 128 Calories 7.2g fat 10g protein

2. Morning Pizza with Sprouts

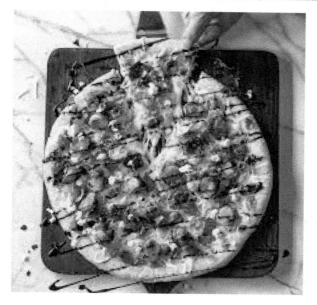

Preparation Time: 15 minutes

Cooking Time: 20 minutes

Servings: 6

Ingredients

- ½ cup wheat flour, whole grain

- 2 tablespoons butter, softened

- ¼ teaspoon baking powder

- ¾ teaspoon salt

- 5 oz chicken fillet, boiled

- 2 oz Cheddar cheese, shredded

- 1 teaspoon tomato sauce

- 1 oz bean sprouts

Directions

1. Make the pizza crust: mix up together wheat flour, butter, baking powder, and salt. Knead the soft and non-sticky dough. Add more wheat flour if needed.

2. Leave the dough for 10 minutes to chill.

3. Then place the dough on the baking paper. Cover it with the second baking paper sheet.

4. Roll up the dough with the help of the rolling pin to get the round pizza crust.

5. After this, remove the upper baking paper sheet.

6. Transfer the pizza crust in the tray.

7. Spread the crust with tomato sauce.

8. Then shred the chicken fillet and arrange it over the pizza crust.

9. Add shredded Cheddar cheese.

10. Bake pizza for 20 minutes at 355F.

11. Then top the cooked pizza with bean sprouts.

Nutrition: 157 Calories 8.8g fat 10.5g protein

3. Banana Quinoa

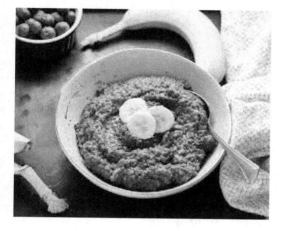

Preparation Time: 10 minutes

Cooking Time: 12 minutes

Servings: 4

Ingredients

- 1 cup quinoa

- 2 cup milk

- 1 teaspoon vanilla extract

- 1 teaspoon honey

- 2 bananas, sliced

- ¼ teaspoon ground cinnamon

Directions

1. Pour milk in the saucepan and add quinoa.

2. Close the lid and cook it over the medium heat for 12 minutes or until quinoa will absorb all liquid.

3. Then chill the quinoa for 10-15 minutes and place in the serving mason jars.

4. Add honey, vanilla extract, and ground cinnamon.

5. Stir well.

6. Top quinoa with banana and stirs it before serving.

Nutrition: 279 Calories 5.3g fat 10.7g protein

4. Avocado Milk Shake

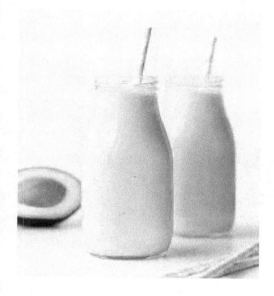

Preparation Time: 10 minutes

Cooking Time: 0 minute

Servings: 2

Ingredients

- 1 avocado, peeled, pitted
- 2 tablespoons of liquid honey
- ½ teaspoon vanilla extract
- ½ cup heavy cream
- 1 cup milk
- 1/3 cup ice cubes

Directions

1. Chop the avocado and put in the food processor.

2. Add liquid honey, vanilla extract, heavy cream, milk, and ice cubes.

3. Blend the mixture until it smooth.

4. Pour the cooked milkshake in the serving glasses.

Nutrition: 291 Calories 22g fat 4.4g protein

5. Egg Casserole with Paprika

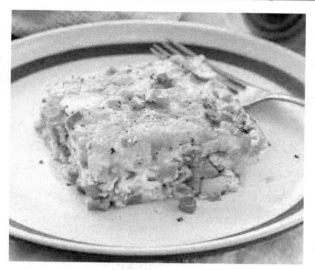

Preparation Time: 10 minutes

Cooking Time: 28 minutes

Servings: 4

Ingredients

- 2 eggs, beaten
- 1 red bell pepper, chopped
- 1 chili pepper, chopped
- ½ red onion, diced
- 1 teaspoon canola oil
- ½ teaspoon salt
- 1 teaspoon paprika

- 1 tablespoon fresh cilantro, chopped

- 1 garlic clove, diced

- 1 teaspoon butter, softened

- ¼ teaspoon chili flakes

Directions

1. Brush the casserole mold with canola oil and pour beaten eggs inside.
2. After this, toss the butter in the skillet and melt it over the medium heat.
3. Add chili pepper and red bell pepper.
4. After this, add red onion and cook the vegetables for 7-8 minutes over the medium heat. Stir them from time to time.
5. Transfer the vegetables in the casserole mold.
6. Add salt, paprika, cilantro, diced garlic, and chili flakes. Stir mildly with spatula to get a homogenous mixture.
7. Bake the casserole for 20 minutes at 355F in the oven.
8. Then chill the meal well and cut into servings. Transfer the casserole in the serving plates with the help of the spatula.

Nutrition: 68 Calories 4.5g fat 3.4g protein

6. Cauliflower Fritters

Preparation Time: 10 minutes

Cooking Time: 10 minutes

Servings: 4

Ingredients

- 1 cup cauliflower, shredded
- 1 egg, beaten
- 1 tablespoon wheat flour, whole grain
- 1 oz Parmesan, grated
- ½ teaspoon ground black pepper
- 1 tablespoon canola oil

Directions

1. In the mixing bowl mix up together shredded cauliflower and egg.
2. Add wheat flour, grated Parmesan, and ground black pepper.
3. Stir the mixture with the help of the fork until it is homogenous and smooth.
4. Pour canola oil in the skillet and bring it to boil.
5. Make the fritters from the cauliflower mixture with the help of the fingertips or use spoon and transfer in the hot oil.

6.   Roast the fritters for 4 minutes from each side over the medium-low heat.

Nutrition: 167 Calories 12.3g fat 8.8g protein

7. Creamy Oatmeal with Figs

Preparation Time: 10 minutes

Cooking Time: 20 minutes

Servings: 5

Ingredients

- 2 cups oatmeal
- 1 ½ cup milk
- 1 tablespoon butter
- 3 figs, chopped
- 1 tablespoon honey

Directions

1. Pour milk in the saucepan.
2. Add oatmeal and close the lid.
3. Cook the oatmeal for 15 minutes over the medium-low heat.
4. Then add chopped figs and honey.
5. Add butter and mix up the oatmeal well.
6. Cook it for 5 minutes more.
7. Close the lid and let the cooked breakfast rest for 10 minutes before serving.

Nutrition: 222 Calories 6g fat 7.1g protein

8. Baked Oatmeal with Cinnamon

Preparation Time: 10 minutes

Cooking Time: 25 minutes

Servings: 4

Ingredients

- 1 cup oatmeal
- 1/3 cup milk
- 1 pear, chopped
- 1 teaspoon vanilla extract
- 1 tablespoon Splenda
- 1 teaspoon butter
- ½ teaspoon ground cinnamon
- 1 egg, beaten

Directions

1. In the big bowl mix up together oatmeal, milk, egg, vanilla extract, Splenda, and ground cinnamon.
2. Melt butter and add it in the oatmeal mixture.
3. Then add chopped pear and stir it well.

4. Transfer the oatmeal mixture in the casserole mold and flatten gently. Cover it with the foil and secure edges.
5. Bake the oatmeal for 25 minutes at 350F.

Nutrition: 151 Calories 3.9g fat 4.9g protein

9. Almond Chia Porridge

Preparation Time: 10 minutes

Cooking Time: 30 minutes

Servings: 4

Ingredients

- 3 cups organic almond milk
- 1/3 cup chia seeds, dried
- 1 teaspoon vanilla extract
- 1 tablespoon honey
- ¼ teaspoon ground cardamom

Directions

1. Pour almond milk in the saucepan and bring it to boil.
2. Then chill the almond milk to the room temperature (or appx. For 10-15 minutes).
3. Add vanilla extract, honey, and ground cardamom. Stir well.
4. After this, add chia seeds and stir again.
5. Close the lid and let chia seeds soak the liquid for 20-25 minutes.
6. Transfer the cooked porridge into the serving ramekins.

Nutrition: 150 Calories 7.3g fat 3.7g protein

10. Cocoa Oatmeal

Preparation Time: 10 minutes

Cooking Time: 15 minutes

Servings: 2

Ingredients

- 1 ½ cup oatmeal

- 1 tablespoon cocoa powder

- ½ cup heavy cream

- ¼ cup of water

- 1 teaspoon vanilla extract

- 1 tablespoon butter

- 2 tablespoons Splenda

Directions

1. Mix up together oatmeal with cocoa powder and Splenda.
2. Transfer the mixture in the saucepan.
3. Add vanilla extract, water, and heavy cream. Stir it gently with the help of the spatula.
4. Close the lid and cook it for 10-15 minutes over the medium-low heat.

5.   Remove the cooked cocoa oatmeal from the heat and add butter. Stir it well.

Nutrition: 230 Calories 10.6g fat 4.6g protein

APPETIZERS AND SNACKS

11. Chickpeas and Red Pepper Hummus

Preparation Time: 10 minutes

Cooking Time: 0 minute

Servings: 6

Ingredients:

- 6 ounces roasted red peppers, peeled and chopped
- 16 ounces canned chickpeas, drained and rinsed
- ¼ cup Greek yogurt
- 3 tablespoons tahini paste
- Juice of 1 lemon
- 3 garlic cloves, minced
- 1 tablespoon olive oil
- A pinch of salt and black pepper
- 1 tablespoon parsley, chopped

Directions:

1. In your food processor, combine the red peppers with the rest of the ingredients except the oil and the parsley and pulse well. Add the oil, pulse again, divide into cups, sprinkle the parsley on top and serve as a party spread.

Nutrition 255 Calories 11.4g Fat 17.4g Carbohydrates 6.5g Protein

12. White Bean Dip

Preparation Time: 10 minutes

Cooking Time: 0 minute

Servings: 4

Ingredients:

- 15 ounces canned white beans, drained and rinsed
- 6 ounces canned artichoke hearts, drained and quartered
- 4 garlic cloves, minced
- 1 tablespoon basil, chopped
- 2 tablespoons olive oil
- Juice of ½ lemon
- Zest of ½ lemon, grated
- Salt and black pepper to the taste

Directions:

1. In your food processor, combine the beans with the artichokes and the rest of the ingredients except the oil and pulse well. Add the oil gradually, pulse the mix again, divide into cups and serve as a party dip.

Nutrition 27 Calories 11.7g Fat 18.5g Carbohydrates 16.5g Protein

13. Hummus with Ground Lamb

Preparation Time: 10 minutes

Cooking Time: 15 minutes

Servings: 8

Ingredients:

- 10 ounces hummus
- 12 ounces lamb meat, ground
- ½ cup pomegranate seeds
- ¼ cup parsley, chopped
- 1 tablespoon olive oil
- Pita chips for serving

Directions:

1. Preheat pan over medium-high heat, cook the meat, and brown for 15 minutes stirring often. Spread the hummus on a platter, spread the ground lamb all over, also spread the pomegranate seeds and the parsley and serve with pita chips as a snack.

Nutrition 133 Calories 9.7g Fat 6.4g Carbohydrates 5.4g Protein

14. Eggplant Dip

Preparation Time: 10 minutes

Cooking Time: 40 minutes

Servings: 4

Ingredients:

- 1 eggplant, poked with a fork
- 2 tablespoons tahini paste
- 2 tablespoons lemon juice
- 2 garlic cloves, minced
- 1 tablespoon olive oil
- Salt and black pepper to the taste
- 1 tablespoon parsley, chopped

Directions:

1. Put the eggplant in a roasting pan, bake at 400 degrees F for 40 minutes, cool down, peel and transfer to your food processor. Blend the rest of the ingredients except the parsley, pulse well, divide into small bowls and serve as an appetizer with the parsley sprinkled on top.

Nutrition 121 Calories 4.3g Fat 1.4g Carbohydrates 4.3g Protein

15. Veggie Fritters

Preparation Time: 10 minutes

Cooking Time: 10 minutes

Servings: 8

Ingredients:

- 2 garlic cloves, minced
- 2 yellow onions, chopped
- 4 scallions, chopped
- 2 carrots, grated
- 2 teaspoons cumin, ground
- ½ teaspoon turmeric powder
- Salt and black pepper to the taste
- ¼ teaspoon coriander, ground
- 2 tablespoons parsley, chopped
- ¼ teaspoon lemon juice
- ½ cup almond flour
- 2 beets, peeled and grated
- 2 eggs, whisked
- ¼ cup tapioca flour
- 3 tablespoons olive oil

Directions:

1. In a bowl, combine the garlic with the onions, scallions and the rest of the ingredients except the oil, stir well and shape medium fritters out of this mix.

2. Preheat pan over medium-high heat, place the fritters, cook for 5 minutes on each side, arrange on a platter and serve.

Nutrition 209 Calories 11.2g Fat 4.4g Carbohydrates 4.8g Protein

16. Bulgur Lamb Meatballs

Preparation Time: 10 minutes

Cooking Time: 15 minutes

Servings: 6

Ingredients:

- 1 and ½ cups Greek yogurt
- ½ teaspoon cumin, ground
- 1 cup cucumber, shredded
- ½ teaspoon garlic, minced
- A pinch of salt and black pepper
- 1 cup bulgur
- 2 cups water
- 1-pound lamb, ground
- ¼ cup parsley, chopped
- ¼ cup shallots, chopped
- ½ teaspoon allspice, ground
- ½ teaspoon cinnamon powder
- 1 tablespoon olive oil

Directions:

1. Mix the bulgur with the water, cover the bowl, leave aside for 10 minutes, drain and transfer to a bowl. Add the meat, the yogurt and the rest of the ingredients except the oil, stir well and shape medium meatballs out of this mix. Preheat pan over medium-high heat, place the meatballs, cook them for 7 minutes on each

side, arrange them all on a platter and serve as an appetizer.

Nutrition   300 Calories 9.6g Fat 22.6g Carbohydrates 6.6g Protein

17. Cucumber Bites

Preparation Time: 10 minutes

Cooking Time: 0 minute

Servings: 12

Ingredients:

- 1 English cucumber, sliced into 32 rounds
- 10 ounces hummus
- 16 cherry tomatoes, halved
- 1 tablespoon parsley, chopped
- 1-ounce feta cheese, crumbled

Directions:

1. Spread the hummus on each cucumber round, divide the tomato halves on each, sprinkle the cheese and parsley on to and serve as an appetizer.

Nutrition 162 Calories 3.4g Fat 6.4g Carbohydrates 2.4g Protein

18. Stuffed Avocado

Preparation Time: 10 minutes

Cooking Time: 0 minute

Servings: 2

Ingredients:

- 1 avocado, halved and pitted
- 10 ounces canned tuna, drained
- 2 tablespoons sun-dried tomatoes, chopped
- 1 and ½ tablespoon basil pesto
- 2 tablespoons black olives, pitted and chopped
- Salt and black pepper to the taste
- 2 teaspoons pine nuts, toasted and chopped
- 1 tablespoon basil, chopped

Directions:

1. Mix the tuna with the sun-dried tomatoes and the rest of the ingredients except the avocado and stir. Stuff the avocado halves with the tuna mix and serve as an appetizer.

Nutrition 233 Calories 9g Fat 11.4g Carbohydrates 5.6g Protein

19. Wrapped Plums

Preparation Time: 5 minutes

Cooking Time: 0 minute

Servings: 8

Ingredients:

- 2 ounces prosciutto, cut into 16 pieces
- 4 plums, quartered
- 1 tablespoon chives, chopped
- A pinch of red pepper flakes, crushed

Directions:

1. Wrap each plum quarter in a prosciutto slice, arrange them all on a platter, sprinkle the chives and pepper flakes all over and serve.

Nutrition 30 Calories 1g Fat 4g Carbohydrates 2g Protein

20. Guaca Egg Scramble

Preparation Time: 8 minutes

Cooking Time: 15 minutes

Servings: 4

Ingredients

- 4 eggs, beaten
- 1 white onion, diced
- 1 tablespoon avocado oil
- 1 avocado, finely chopped
- ½ teaspoon chili flakes
- 1 oz Cheddar cheese, shredded
- ½ teaspoon salt
- 1 tablespoon fresh parsley

Directions:

1. Pour avocado oil in the skillet and bring it to boil. Then add diced onion and roast it until it is light brown. Meanwhile, mix up together chili flakes, beaten eggs, and salt.
2. Fill the egg mixture over the cooked onion and cook the mixture for 1 minute over the medium heat. After this, scramble the eggs well with the help of the fork or spatula. Cook the eggs until they are solid but soft.

3. After this, add chopped avocado and shredded cheese. Stir the scramble well and transfer in the serving plates. Sprinkle the meal with fresh parsley.

Nutrition   236 Calories   20g Fat   4g Carbohydrates 8.6g Protein

MAIN DISH

21. Garlic-Herb Rice

Preparation Time: 10 minutes

Cooking Time: 30 minutes

Servings: 4

Ingredients

- Extra-virgin olive oil – ½ cup, divided
- Large garlic cloves – 5, minced
- Brown jasmine rice – 2 cups
- Water – 4 cups
- Sea salt – 1 tsp.
- Black pepper – 1 tsp.
- Chopped fresh chives – 3 tbsp.
- Chopped fresh parsley – 2 tbsp.
- Chopped fresh basil – 1 tbsp.

Directions:

1. In a saucepan, add ¼-cup olive oil, garlic, and rice. Stir and heat over medium heat. Stir in the water, sea salt, and black pepper. Next, mix again.
2. Boil and lower the heat. Simmer, uncovered, stirring occasionally.

3. When the water is almost absorbed, mix the remaining ¼-cup olive oil, along with the basil, parsley, and chives.

4. Stir until the herbs are incorporated and all the water is absorbed.

Nutrition 304 Calories 25.8g Fat 19.3g Carb 2g Protein

22. Mediterranean Rice Salad

Preparation Time: 10 minutes

Cooking Time: 25 minutes

Servings: 4

Ingredients

- Extra virgin olive oil – ½ cup, divided
- Long-grain brown rice – 1 cup
- Water – 2 cups
- Fresh lemon juice – ¼ cup
- Garlic clove – 1, minced
- Minced fresh rosemary – 1 tsp.
- Minced fresh mint – 1 tsp.
- Belgian endives – 3, chopped
- Red bell pepper – 1 medium, chopped
- Hothouse cucumber – 1, chopped
- Chopped whole green onion – ½ cup
- Chopped Kalamata olives – ½ cup
- Red pepper flakes – ¼ tsp.
- Crumbled feta cheese – ¾ cup
- Sea salt and black pepper

Directions:

1. Heat ¼-cup olive oil, rice, and a pinch of salt in a saucepan over low heat. Stir to coat the rice. Add the water and let simmer until the water is absorbed.

Stirring occasionally. Fill in the rice into a big bowl and cool.

2. Scourge remaining ¼ cup olive oil, red pepper flakes, olives, green onion, cucumber, bell pepper, endives, mint, rosemary, garlic, and lemon juice.

3. Place the rice to the mixture and toss to combine. Gently mix in the feta cheese.

4. Taste and adjust the seasoning. Serve.

Nutrition   415 Calories 34g Fat 28.3g Carbohydrates 7g Protein

23. Fresh Bean and Tuna Salad

Preparation Time: 5 minutes

Cooking Time: 20 minutes

Servings: 6

Ingredients

- Shelled (shucked) fresh beans – 2 cups
- Bay leaves – 2
- Extra-virgin olive oil – 3 tbsp.
- Red wine vinegar – 1 tbsp.
- Salt and black pepper
- Best-quality tuna - 1 (6-ounce) can, packed in olive oil
- Salted capers – 1 tbsp. soaked and dried
- Finely minced flat-leaf parsley – 2 tbsp.
- Red onion – 1, sliced

Directions:

1. Boil lightly salted water in a pot. Add the beans and bay leaves; next, cook for 15 to 20 minutes, or until the beans are tender but still firm. Drain, discard aromatics, and transfer to a bowl.

2. Immediately dress the beans with vinegar and oil. Add the salt and black pepper. Mix well and adjust seasoning. Drain the tuna and flake the tuna flesh into

the bean salad. Add the parsley and capers. Toss to mix and scatter the red onion slices over the top. Serve.

Nutrition 85 Calories 7.1g Fat 4.7g Carbohydrates 1.8g Protein

24. Baked Balsamic Fish

Preparation Time: 10 minutes

Cooking Time: 10 minutes

Servings: 4

Ingredients:

- 1 tablespoon balsamic vinegar
- 2 ½ cups green beans
- 1-pint cherry or grape tomatoes
- 4 (4-ounce each) fish fillets, such as cod or tilapia
- 2 tablespoons olive oil

Directions:

1. Preheat an oven to 400 degrees. Grease two baking sheets with some olive oil or olive oil spray. Arrange 2 fish fillets on each sheet. In a mixing bowl, pour olive oil and vinegar. Combine to mix well with each other.
2. Mix green beans and tomatoes. Combine to mix well with each other. Combine both mixtures well with each other. Add mixture equally over fish fillets. Bake for 6-8 minutes, until fish opaque and easy to flake. Serve warm.

Nutrition 229 Calories 13g Fat 8g Carbohydrates 2.5g Protein

25. Cod-Mushroom Soup

Preparation Time: 10 minutes

Cooking Time: 20 minutes

Servings: 6

Ingredients:

- 2 tablespoons extra-virgin olive oil
- 2 garlic cloves, minced
- 1 can tomato
- 2 cups chopped onion
- ¾ teaspoon smoked paprika
- a (12-ounce) jar roasted red peppers
- 1/3 cup dry red wine
- ¼ teaspoon kosher or sea salt
- ¼ teaspoon black pepper
- 1 cup black olives
- 1 ½ pounds cod fillets, cut into 1-inch pieces
- 3 cups sliced mushrooms

Directions:

1. Get medium-large cooking pot, warm up oil over medium heat. Add onions and stir-cook for 4 minutes. Add garlic and smoked paprika; cook for 1 minute, stirring often. Add tomatoes with juice, roasted peppers, olives, wine, pepper, and salt; stir gently. Boil mixture. Add the cod and mushrooms; turn down heat

to medium. Close and cook until the cod is easy to flake, stir in between. Serve warm.

Nutrition 238 Calories 7g Fat 15g Carbohydrates 3.5g Protein

26. Mediterranean-Spiced Swordfish

Preparation Time: 10 minutes

Cooking Time: 15 minutes

Servings: 4

Ingredients:

- 4 (7 ounces each) swordfish steaks
- 1/2 teaspoon ground black pepper
- 12 cloves of garlic, peeled
- 3/4 teaspoon salt
- 1 1/2 teaspoon ground cumin
- 1 teaspoon paprika
- 1 teaspoon coriander
- 3 tablespoons lemon juice
- 1/3 cup olive oil

Directions:

1. Using food processor, incorporate all the ingredients except for swordfish. Seal the lid and blend to make a smooth mixture. Pat dry fish steaks; coat equally with the prepared spice mixture.
2. Situate them over an aluminum foil, cover and refrigerator for 1 hour. Prep a griddle pan over high heat, cook oil. Put fish steaks; stir-cook for 5-6 minutes per side until cooked through and evenly browned. Serve warm.

Nutrition 275 Calories 17g Fat 5g Carbohydrates 0.5g Protein

27. Anchovy-Parmesan Pasta

Preparation Time: 10 minutes

Cooking Time: 20 minutes

Servings: 4

Ingredients:

- 4 anchovy fillets, packed in olive oil
- ½ pound broccoli, cut into 1-inch florets
- 2 cloves garlic, sliced
- 1-pound whole-wheat penne
- 2 tablespoons olive oil
- ¼ cup Parmesan cheese, grated
- Salt and black pepper, to taste
- Red pepper flakes, to taste

Directions:

1. Cook pasta as directed over pack; drain and set aside. Take a medium saucepan or skillet, add oil. Heat over medium heat.
2. Add anchovies, broccoli, and garlic, and stir-cook until veggies turn tender for 4-5 minutes. Take off heat; mix in the pasta. Serve warm with Parmesan cheese, red pepper flakes, salt, and black pepper sprinkled on top.

Nutrition 328 Calories 8g Fat 35g Carbohydrates 7g Protein

28. Garlic-Shrimp Pasta

Preparation Time: 10 minutes

Cooking Time: 15 minutes

Servings: 4

Ingredients:

- 1-pound shrimp, peeled and deveined
- 3 garlic cloves, minced
- 1 onion, finely chopped
- 1 package whole wheat or bean pasta of your choice
- 4 tablespoons olive oil
- Salt and black pepper, to taste
- ¼ cup basil, cut into strips
- ¾ cup chicken broth, low-sodium

Directions:

1. Cook pasta as directed over pack; rinse and set aside. Get medium saucepan, add oil then warm up over medium heat. Add onion, garlic and stir-cook until become translucent and fragrant for 3 minutes.
2. Add shrimp, black pepper (ground) and salt; stir-cook for 3 minutes until shrimps are opaque. Add broth and simmer for 2-3 more minutes. Add pasta in serving plates; add shrimp mixture over; serve warm with basil on top.

Nutrition 605 Calories 17g Fat 53g Carbohydrates 19g Protein

VEGETABLES AND SIDE DISHES

29. Tomato-Garlic Spanish Rice

Preparation Time: 10 minutes

Cooking Time: 35 minutes

Serving: 4

Ingredients:

- ¼ cup olive oil

- 1 small onion

- 1 red bell pepper

- 1½ cups white rice

- 1 teaspoon sweet paprika

- ½ teaspoon ground cumin

- ½ teaspoon ground coriander

- 1 garlic clove, minced

- 3 tablespoons tomato paste

- 3 cups vegetable broth

- 1/8 teaspoon salt

Direction:

1. Using big heavy-bottomed skillet over medium heat, heat the olive oil.

2. Stir in the onion and red bell pepper. Cook for 5 minutes or until softened.

3. Add the rice, paprika, cumin, and coriander and cook for 2 minutes, stirring often.

4. Add the garlic, tomato paste, vegetable broth, and salt. Stir and season with more salt, as needed.

5. Increase the heat to bring the mixture to a boil. Reduce the heat to low, cover the skillet, and simmer for 20 minutes.

6. Let the rice rest, covered, for 5 minutes before serving.

Nutrition: 414 calories 14g fat 6g protein

30. Zucchini and Rice with Tzatziki Sauce

Preparation Time: 20 minutes

Cooking Time: 35 minutes

Serving: 4

Ingredients:

- ¼ cup olive oil

- 1 onion

- 3 zucchinis

- 1 cup vegetable broth

- ½ cup chopped fresh dill

- 1 cup short-grain rice

- 2 tablespoons pine nuts

- 1 cup Tzatziki Sauce, Plain Yogurt

Direction:

1. Using heavy-bottomed pot over medium heat, heat the olive oil.

2. Mix in onion, turn the heat to medium-low, and sauté for 5 minutes.

3. Stir in zucchini and cook for 2 minutes more.

4. Fill in the vegetable broth and dill and season with salt and pepper. Increase the heat to medium and bring the mixture to a boil.

5. Mix in the rice and let it boil. Set to very low heat, cover the pot, and cook for 15 minutes. Remove from the heat and let the rice rest, covered, for 10 minutes.

6. Ladle the rice onto a serving platter, sprinkle with the pine nuts, and serve with tzatziki sauce.

Nutrition: 414 calories 17g fat 11g protein

31. Rosemary, Garlic Aioli and Cannellini Beans

Preparation Time: 10 minutes

Cooking Time: 10 minutes

Serving: 4

Ingredients:

- 4 cups cooked cannellini beans
- 4 cups water
- ½ teaspoon salt
- 3 tablespoons olive oil
- 2 tablespoons chopped fresh rosemary
- ½ cup Garlic Aioli

Direction:

1. Using medium saucepan over medium heat, mix cannellini beans, water, and salt. Bring to a boil. Cook for 5 minutes. Drain.

2. In a skillet over medium heat, cook olive oil.

3. Add the beans. Stir in the rosemary and aioli. Switch heat to medium-low and cook, stirring, just to heat through. Season with pepper and serve.

Nutrition: 545 calories 36g fat 15g protein

32. Jeweled Basmati Rice

Preparation Time: 15 minutes

Cooking Time: 30 minutes

Serving: 6

Ingredients:

- ½ cup olive oil, divided
- 1 onion, finely chopped
- 1 garlic clove, minced
- ½ teaspoon fresh ginger
- 4½ cups water
- 1 teaspoon salt
- 1 teaspoon ground turmeric
- 2 cups basmati rice
- 1 cup fresh sweet peas
- 2 carrots
- ½ cup dried cranberries
- Grated zest of 1 orange
- 1/8 teaspoon cayenne pepper
- ¼ cup slivered almonds

Direction:

1. Using huge heavy-bottomed pot over medium heat, heat ¼ cup of olive oil.

2. Stir in onion and cook for 4 minutes. Add the garlic and ginger and cook for 1 minute more.

3. Pour in the water, ¾ teaspoon of salt, and the turmeric. Bring the mixture to a boil. Mix in the rice and boil. Select heat to low, cover the pot, and cook for 15 minutes. Turn off the heat. Let the rice rest on the burner, covered, for 10 minutes.

4. Meanwhile, using medium sauté pan or skillet over medium-low heat, cook remaining ¼ cup of olive oil. Stir in the peas and carrots. Cook for 5 minutes.

5. Drizzle cranberries and orange zest. Season with the remaining ¼ teaspoon of salt and the cayenne. Cook for 1 to 2 minutes.

6. Ladle the rice onto a serving platter. Top with the peas and carrots and sprinkle with the toasted almonds.

Nutrition: 460 calories 19g fat 7g protein

33. Cheese Asparagus Risotto

Preparation Time: 15 minutes

Cooking Time: 30 minutes

Serving: 4

Ingredients:

- 5 cups vegetable broth
- 3 tablespoons unsalted butter
- 1 tablespoon olive oil
- 1 small onion, chopped
- 1½ cups Arborio rice
- 1-pound fresh asparagus
- ¼ cup grated Parmesan cheese

Direction:

1. In a saucepan over medium heat, bring the vegetable broth to a boil. Switch heat to low and keep the broth at a steady simmer.

2. In a 4-quart heavy-bottomed saucepan over medium heat, melt 2 tablespoons of butter with the olive oil. Add the onion and cook for 2 to 3 minutes.

3. Add the rice and stir with a wooden spoon while cooking for 1 minute.

4. Stir in ½ cup of warm broth. Cook, stirring often, for about 5 minutes until the broth is completely absorbed.

5. Add the asparagus stalks and another ½ cup of broth. Cook, stirring often, until the liquid is absorbed. Continue adding the broth, ½ cup at a time, and cooking until it is completely absorbed before adding the next ½ cup. Stir frequently to prevent sticking. After about 20 minutes, the rice should be cooked but still firm.

6. Add the asparagus tips, the remaining 1 tablespoon of butter, and the Parmesan cheese. Stir vigorously to combine.

7. Remove from the heat, top with additional Parmesan cheese, if desired, and serve immediately.

Nutrition: 434 calories 14g fat 10g protein

34. Spanish Vegan Paella

Preparation Time: 25 minutes

Cooking Time: 45 minutes

Serving: 6

Ingredients:

- ¼ cup olive oil
- 1 large sweet onion
- 1 large red bell pepper
- 1 large green bell pepper
- 3 garlic cloves
- 1 teaspoon smoked paprika
- 5 saffron threads
- 1 zucchini, cut into ½-inch cubes
- 4 large ripe tomatoes
- 1½ cups short-grain Spanish rice
- 3 cups vegetable broth, warmed

Direction:

1. Preheat the oven to 350°F.

2. Using oven-safe skillet over medium heat, heat the olive oil.

3. Stir in onion and red and green bell peppers and cook for 10 minutes.

4. Mix in the garlic, paprika, saffron threads, zucchini, and tomatoes. Turn the heat to medium-low and cook for 10 minutes.

5. Pour in the rice and vegetable broth. Increase the heat to bring the paella to a boil. Reduce the heat to medium-low and cook for 15 minutes. Cover the pan with aluminum foil and put it in the oven.

6. Bake for 10 minutes.

Nutrition: 288 calories 10g fat 5g protein

35. Japanese Eggplant Casserole

Preparation Time: 30 minutes

Cooking Time: 35 minutes

Serving: 4

Ingredients:

For sauce

- ½ cup olive oil
- 1 small onion
- 4 garlic cloves
- 6 ripe tomatoes
- 2 tablespoons tomato paste
- 1 teaspoon dried oregano
- ¼ teaspoon ground nutmeg

For casserole

- 4 (6-inch) Japanese eggplants
- 2 tablespoons olive oil
- 1 cup cooked rice
- 2 tablespoons pine nuts
- 1 cup water

Direction:

For sauce

1. Using heavy-bottomed saucepan over medium heat, heat the olive oil. Stir in onion and cook for 5 minutes.

2. Mix in the garlic, tomatoes, tomato paste, oregano, nutmeg, and cumin. Bring to a boil. Close, switch heat to low, and simmer for 10 minutes. Remove and set aside.

For casserole

3. Prep the broiler.

4. While the sauce simmers, rub eggplant with the olive oil and situate them on a baking sheet. Broil for about 5 minutes until golden. Remove and let cool.

5. Switch the oven to 375°F. Arrange the cooled eggplant, cut-side up, in a 9-by-13-inch baking dish. Gently spoon out some flesh to make room for the stuffing.

6. Incorporate half the tomato sauce, the cooked rice, and pine nuts. Fill each eggplant half with the rice mixture.

7. Mix remaining tomato sauce and water. Pour over the eggplant.

8. Bake for 20 minutes.

Nutrition: 453 calories 39g fat 6g protein

36. Veggie Couscous

Preparation Time: 15 minutes

Cooking Time: 45 minutes

Serving: 8

Ingredient

- ¼ cup olive oil

- 1 onion

- 4 garlic cloves

- 2 jalapeño peppers

- ½ tsp. ground cumin

- ½ tsp. ground coriander

- 1 (28-oz) can crushed tomatoes

- 2 tbsp. tomato paste

- 1/8 tsp. salt

- 2 bay leaves

- 11 cups water

- 4 carrots, cut into 2-inch pieces

- 2 zucchinis

- 1 acorn squash

- 1 (15-oz) can chickpeas

- ¼ cup Preserved Lemons

- 3 cups couscous

Direction:

1. Using big heavy-bottomed pot over medium heat, heat the olive oil. Stir in the onion and cook for 4 minutes. Stir in the garlic, jalapeños, cumin, and coriander. Cook for 1 minute.

2. Mix in tomatoes, tomato paste, salt, bay leaves, and 8 cups of water. Bring the mixture to a boil.

3. Stir in carrots, zucchini, and acorn squash and return to a boil. Reduce the heat slightly, cover, and cook for about 20 minutes until the vegetables are tender but not mushy. Remove 2 cups of the cooking liquid and set aside. Season as needed.

4. Mix in chickpeas and preserved lemons (if using). Cook for 2 to 3 minutes, and turn off the heat.

5. Using medium pan, bring the remaining 3 cups of water to a boil over high heat. Stir in the couscous, cover, and turn off the heat. Let the couscous rest for 10 minutes. Drizzle with 1 cup of reserved cooking liquid. Using a fork, fluff the couscous.

6. Drizzle with the remaining cooking liquid. Remove the vegetables from the pot and arrange on top. Serve the remaining stew in a separate bowl.

Nutrition: 415 calories 7g fat 14g protein

37. Egyptian Koshari

Preparation Time: 25 minutes

Cooking Time: 80 minutes

Serving: 8

Ingredients:

For sauce

- 2 tablespoons olive oil

- 2 garlic cloves, minced

- 1 (16-ounce) can tomato sauce

- ¼ cup white vinegar

- ¼ cup Harissa, or store-bought

- 1/8 teaspoon salt

For rice

- 1 cup olive oil

- 2 onions, thinly sliced

- 2 cups dried brown lentils

- 4 quarts plus ½ cup water

- 2 cups short-grain rice

- 1 teaspoon salt

- 1-pound short elbow pasta

- 1 (15-ounce) can chickpeas

Direction:

For sauce

1. In a saucepan over medium heat, heat the olive oil.

2. Stir in garlic and cook for 1 minute.

3. Stir in the tomato sauce, vinegar, harissa, and salt. Increase the heat to bring the sauce to a boil. Adjust the heat to low and cook for 20 minutes or until the sauce has thickened. Remove and set aside.

For rice

4. Prep the plate with paper towels and put aside.

5. In a large pan over medium heat, heat the olive oil.

6. Add the onions and cook for 7 to 10 minutes, stirring often, until crisp and golden. Transfer the onions to the prepared plate and set aside. Reserve 2 tablespoons of the cooking oil. Reserve the pan.

7. Using big pot over high heat, mix the lentils and 4 cups of water. Bring to a boil and cook for 20 minutes. Drain, situate to a bowl, and pour in the reserved 2 tablespoons of cooking oil. Set aside. Reserve the pot.

8. Place the pan you used to fry the onions over medium-high heat and add the rice, 4½ cups of water, and sprinkle salt to it. Bring to a boil then switch heat to low, then cook for 20 minutes. Turn off the heat and let the rice rest for 10 minutes.6.

9. In the pot used to cook the lentils, bring the remaining 8 cups of water, salted, to a boil over high heat. Stir in the pasta and cook for 7 minutes or according to the package instructions. Drain and set aside.

10. To assemble: Spoon the rice onto a serving platter. Top it with the lentils, chickpeas, and pasta. Drizzle with the hot tomato sauce and sprinkle with the crispy fried onions.

Nutrition: 668 calories 13g fat 25g protein

38. Tomatoes and Chickpeas Bulgur

Preparation Time: 10 minutes

Cooking Time: 35 minutes

Serving: 6

Ingredients:

- ½ cup olive oil

- 1 onion, chopped

- 6 tomatoes

- 2 tablespoons tomato paste

- 2 cups water

- 1 tablespoon Harissa

- 1/8 teaspoon salt

- 2 cups coarse bulgur #3

- 1 (15-ounce) can chickpeas

Direction:

1. Using heavy-bottomed pot over medium heat, heat the olive oil.

2. Cook onion for 5 minutes.

3. Add the tomatoes with their juice and cook for 5 minutes.

4. Stir in the tomato paste, water, harissa, and salt. Bring to a boil.

5. Stir in the bulgur and chickpeas. Return the mixture to a boil. Switch heat to low, cover then cook for 15 minutes. Let rest for 15 minutes before serving.

Nutrition: 413 calories 19g fat 11g protein

SOUP AND STEW RECIPES

39. Sausage Kale Soup with Mushrooms

Preparation Time: 8 minutes

Cooking Time: 70 minutes

Serving: 6

Ingredients:

- 2 cups fresh kale
- 6.5 ounces mushrooms, sliced
- 6 cups chicken bone broth
- 1-pound sausage, cooked and sliced

Directions:

1. Heat chicken broth with two cans of water in a large pot and bring to a boil.

2. Stir in the remaining ingredients and allow the soup to simmer on low heat for about 1 hour.

3. Dish out and serve hot.

Nutrition: 259 Calories 20g Fats 14g Proteins

40. Classic Minestrone

Preparation Time: 12 minutes

Cooking Time: 25 minutes

Serving: 6

Ingredients:

- 2 tablespoons olive oil
- 3 cloves garlic
- 1 onion, diced
- 2 carrots
- 2 stalks celery
- 1 1/2 teaspoons dried basil
- 1 teaspoon dried oregano
- 1/2 teaspoon fennel seed
- 6 cups low sodium chicken broth
- 1 (28-ounce) can tomatoes
- 1 (16-ounce) can kidney beans
- 1 zucchini
- 1 Parmesan rind
- 1 bay leaf

- 1 bunch kale leaves, chopped

- 2 teaspoons red wine vinegar

- 1/3 cup freshly grated Parmesan

- 2 tablespoons chopped fresh parsley leaves

Directions:

1. Preheat olive oil in the insert of the Instant Pot on Sauté mode.

2. Add carrots, celery, and onion, sauté for 3 minutes.

3. Stir in fennel seeds, oregano, and basil. Stir cook for 1 minute.

4. Add stock, beans, tomatoes, parmesan, bay leaf, and zucchini.

5. Secure and seal the Instant Pot lid then select Manual mode to cook for minutes at high pressure.

6. Once done, release the pressure completely then remove the lid.

7. Add kale and let it sit for 2 minutes in the hot soup.

8. Stir in red wine, vinegar, pepper, and salt.

9. Garnish with parsley and parmesan.

Nutrition: 805 Calories 124 Protein 34g Fat

41. Turkey Meatball and Ditalini Soup

Preparation Time: 15 minutes

Cooking Time: 40 minutes

Serving: 4

Ingredients:

meatballs:

- 1 pound 93% lean ground turkey
- 1/3 cup seasoned breadcrumbs
- 3 tablespoons grated Pecorino Romano cheese
- 1 large egg, beaten
- 1 clove crushed garlic
- 1 tablespoon fresh minced parsley
- 1/2 teaspoon kosher salt

Soup:

- 1 teaspoon olive oil
- 1/2 cup onion
- 1/2 cup celery
- 1/2 cup carrot
- 3 cloves garlic

- 1 can San Marzano tomatoes

- 4 cups reduced sodium chicken broth

- 4 torn basil leaves

- 2 bay leaves

- 1 cup ditalini pasta

- 1 cup zucchini, diced small

- Parmesan rind, optional

- Grated parmesan cheese, optional for serving

Directions:

1. Thoroughly combine turkey with egg, garlic, parsley, salt, pecorino and breadcrumbs in a bowl.

2. Make 30 equal sized meatballs out of this mixture.

3. Preheat olive oil in the insert of the Instant Pot on Sauté mode.

4. Sear the meatballs in the heated oil in batches, until brown.

5. Set the meatballs aside in a plate.

6. Add more oil to the insert of the Instant Pot.

7. Stir in carrots, garlic, celery, and onion. Sauté for 4 minutes.

8. Add basil, bay leaves, tomatoes, and Parmesan rind.

9. Return the seared meatballs to the pot along with the broth.

10. Secure and sear the Instant Pot lid and select Manual mode for 15 minutes at high pressure.

11. Once done, release the pressure completely then remove the lid.

12. Add zucchini and pasta, cook it for 4 minutes on Sauté mode.

13. Garnish with cheese and basil.

Nutrition: 261 Calories 37g Protein 7g Fat

42. Mint Avocado Chilled Soup

Preparation Time: 6 minutes

Cooking Time: 0 minutes

Serving: 2

Ingredients:

- 1 cup coconut milk, chilled
- 1 medium ripe avocado
- 1 tablespoon lime juice
- Salt, to taste
- 20 fresh mint leaves

Directions:

1. Put all the ingredients into an immersion blender and blend until a thick mixture is formed.

2. Allow to cool for 10 minutes and serve chilled.

Nutrition: 286 Calories 27g Fats 4.2g Proteins

MEAT RECIPES

43. Double Cheesy Bacon Chicken

Preparation Time: 10 minutes

Cooking Time: 30 minutes

Servings: 4

Ingredients

- 4 oz. or 113 g. Cream Cheese
- 1 c. Cheddar Cheese
- 8 strips Bacon
- Sea salt
- Pepper
- 2 Garlic cloves, finely chopped
- Chicken Breast
- 1 tbsp. Bacon Grease or Butter

Directions:

1. Ready the oven to 400 F/204 C Slice the chicken breasts in half to make them thin
2. Season with salt, pepper, and garlic Grease a baking pan with butter and place chicken breasts into it. Add the cream cheese and cheddar cheese on top of the breasts

3. Add bacon slices as well Place the pan to the oven for 30 minutes Serve hot

Nutrition 610 Calories 32g Fat 3g Carbohydrates 38g Protein

44. Shrimps with Lemon and Pepper

Preparation Time: 10 minutes

Cooking Time: 10 minutes

Servings: 4

Ingredients

- 40 deveined shrimps, peeled
- 6 minced garlic cloves
- Salt and black pepper
- 3 tbsps. olive oil
- ¼ tsp. sweet paprika
- A pinch crushed red pepper flake
- ¼ tsp. grated lemon zest
- 3 tbsps. Sherry or another wine
- 1½ tbsps. sliced chives
- Juice of 1 lemon
-

Directions:

1. Adjust your heat to medium-high and set a pan in place.
2. Add oil and shrimp, sprinkle with pepper and salt and cook for 1 minute Add paprika, garlic and pepper flakes, stir and cook for 1 minute. Gently stir in sherry and allow to cook for an extra minute

3. Take shrimp off the heat, add chives and lemon zest, stir and transfer shrimp to plates. Add lemon juice all over and serve

Nutrition 140 Calories 1g Fat 5g Carbohydrates 18g Protein

45. **Breaded and Spiced Halibut**

Preparation Time: 5 minutes

Cooking Time: 25 minutes

Servings: 4

Ingredients

- ¼ c. chopped fresh chives
- ¼ c. chopped fresh dill
- ¼ tsp. ground black pepper
- ¾ c. panko breadcrumbs
- 1 tbsp. extra-virgin olive oil
- 1 tsp. finely grated lemon zest
- 1 tsp. sea salt
- 1/3 c. chopped fresh parsley
- 4 (6 oz. or 170 g. each) halibut fillets

Directions:

1. In a medium bowl, mix olive oil and the rest ingredients except halibut fillets and breadcrumbs
2. Place halibut fillets into the mixture and marinate for 30 minutes Preheat your oven to 400 F/204 C Set a foil to a baking sheet, grease with cooking spray Dip the fillets to the breadcrumbs and put to the baking sheet Cook in the oven for 20 minutes Serve hot
   Nutrition 667 Calories 24.5g Fat 2g Carbohydrates 54.8g Protein

46. Curry Salmon with Mustard

Preparation Time: 10 minutes

Cooking Time: 20 minutes

Servings: 4

Ingredients

- ¼ tsp. ground red pepper or chili powder
- ¼ tsp. turmeric, ground
- ¼ tsp. salt
- 1 tsp. honey
- ¼ tsp. garlic powder
- 2 tsps. whole grain mustard
- 4 (6 oz. or 170 g. each) salmon fillets

Directions:

1. In a bowl mix mustard and the rest ingredients except salmon   Prep the oven to 350 F. Rub baking dish with cooking spray. Place salmon on baking dish with skin side down and spread evenly mustard mixture on top of fillets Place into the oven and cook for 10-15 minutes or until flaky

Nutrition   324 Calories   18.9g Fat   1.3g Carbohydrates 34g Protein

DESSERT RECIPES

47. Chocolate Rice Pudding

Preparation Time: 10 minutes

Cooking Time: 20 minutes

Servings: 6

Ingredients:

- 2 cups almond milk
- 1 cup long-grain brown rice
- 2 tablespoons Dutch-processed cocoa powder
- ¼ cup maple syrup
- 1 teaspoon vanilla extract
- ½ cup chopped dark chocolate

Directions:

1. Place almond milk, rice, cocoa, maple syrup, and vanilla in the Instant Pot®. Close then select the Manual button, and set time to 20 minutes.
2. When the timer beeps, let pressure release naturally for 15 minutes, then quick-release the remaining pressure. Press the Cancel button and open lid. Serve warm, sprinkled with chocolate.

Nutrition 271 Calories   8g Fat 4g Carbohydrates 3g Protein

48. Fruit Compote

Preparation Time: 10 minutes

Cooking Time: 15 minutes

Servings: 6

Ingredients:

- 1 cup apple juice
- 1 cup dry white wine
- 2 tablespoons honey
- 1 cinnamon stick
- ¼ teaspoon ground nutmeg
- 1 tablespoon grated lemon zest
- 1½ tablespoons grated orange zest
- 3 large apples, peeled, cored, and chopped
- 3 large pears, peeled, cored, and chopped
- ½ cup dried cherries

Directions:

1. Situate all ingredients in the Instant Pot® and stir well. Close and select the Manual button, and allow to sit for 1 minute. When the timer beeps, rapidly-release the pressure until the float valve hit the bottom. Click the Cancel then open lid.
2. Use a slotted spoon to transfer fruit to a serving bowl. Remove and discard cinnamon stick. Press the Sauté button and bring juice in the pot to a boil. Cook, stirring

constantly, until reduced to a syrup that will coat the back of a spoon, about 10 minutes.

3. Stir syrup into fruit mixture. Once cool slightly, then wrap with plastic and chill overnight.

Nutrition 211 Calories   1g Fat 4g Carbohydrates   2g Protein

49. Stuffed Apples

Preparation Time: 10 minutes

Cooking Time: 15 minutes

Servings: 6

Ingredients:

- ½ cup apple juice
- ¼ cup golden raisins
- ¼ cup chopped toasted walnuts
- 2 tablespoons sugar
- ½ teaspoon grated orange zest
- ½ teaspoon ground cinnamon
- 4 large cooking apples
- 4 teaspoons unsalted butter
- 1 cup water

Directions:

1. Put apple juice in a microwave-safe container; heat for 1 minute on high or until steaming and hot. Pour over raisins. Soak raisins for 30 minutes. Drain, reserving apple juice. Add nuts, sugar, orange zest, and cinnamon to raisins and stir to mix.
2. Cut off the top fourth of each apple. Peel the cut portion and chop it, then stir diced apple pieces into raisin mixture. Hollow out and core apples by cutting to, but not through, the bottoms.

3. Situate each apple on a piece of aluminum foil that is large enough to wrap apple completely. Fill apple centers with raisin mixture.
4. Top each with 1 teaspoon butter. Cover the foil around each apple, folding the foil over at the top and then pinching it firmly together.
5. Stir in water to the Instant Pot® and place rack inside. Place apples on the rack. Close lid, set steam release to Sealing, press the Manual, and alarm to 10 minutes.
6. When the timer beeps, quick-release the pressure until the float valve drops and open the lid. Carefully lift apples out of the Instant Pot®. Unwrap and transfer to plates. Serve hot, at room temperature, or cold.

Nutrition 432 Calories   16g Fat   6g Carbohydrates 3g Protein

50. Cinnamon-Stewed Dried Plums with Greek Yogurt

Preparation Time: 10 minutes

Cooking Time: 15 minutes

Servings: 6

Ingredients:

- 3 cups dried plums
- 2 cups water
- 2 tablespoons sugar
- 2 cinnamon sticks
- 3 cups low-fat plain Greek yogurt

Directions:

1. Add dried plums, water, sugar, and cinnamon to the Instant Pot®. Close allow steam release to Sealing, press the Manual button, and start the time to 3 minutes.
2. Once the timer beeps, quick-release the pressure. Click the Cancel button and open. Remove and discard cinnamon sticks. Serve warm over Greek yogurt.

Nutrition 301 Calories   2g Fat 3g Carbohydrates 14g Protein

CONCLUSION

For good health, the Mediterranean diet plan emphasizes consuming healthy food as close to its natural state as possible. Take an apple, for example. An apple is an apple is an apple is an apple is an apple is an apple is an Applesauce is a step back but a world away because the skin is removed, along with all of the fiber, and replaced with sugar. Then there's apple juice, which has even more sugar in it. It's easy to see how even the most basic processing removes the best qualities of a food product.

We tend to prioritize convenience in today's fast-paced society, particularly when it comes to eating. Processed snack foods are more convenient and often more readily available than whole foods, but they're not healthy—and their names, serving sizes, and ingredients are often deceptive. It may be less expensive and more convenient to eat this way, but it comes at a cost to our wellbeing. There's a saying that goes, "Pay it now or pay it later." With obesity and illness on the rise, there's never been a better time to pay attention to how we treat our bodies. We're learning more and more about the advantages of healthy eating, including how it can also help you live longer.

Unrefined, unprocessed foods that foster wellness are at the heart of this initiative. As a dietitian, I believe that food is not only fuel for the body, but also medicine. We would be rewarded with endless health benefits if we adopt a diet like the Mediterranean plan, which is rich in minerals, complex carbohydrates, fruit, vegetables, and healthy fats.

The idea of "eating the rainbow" is well-known. Its value stems from the fact that many produce varieties contain specific nutrients based on their color. Orange-colored produce, such as carrots, sweet potatoes, melon, apricots, and mangos, for example, are high in vitamins A and C, which are essential for vision and immune health. Berries are high in antioxidants and other essential nutrients. Leafy greens are nutritious powerhouses in general. The list could go on and on, but the point is clear: Fill your plate with a rainbow of foods and colors, and you'll reap a slew of benefits.

CPSIA information can be obtained
at www.ICGtesting.com
Printed in the USA
BVHW090734150521
607370BV00012B/2074